Uncovering the Power of Essential Oils

Essential Oil Recipes for Health and Well-being

Contents

Introduction

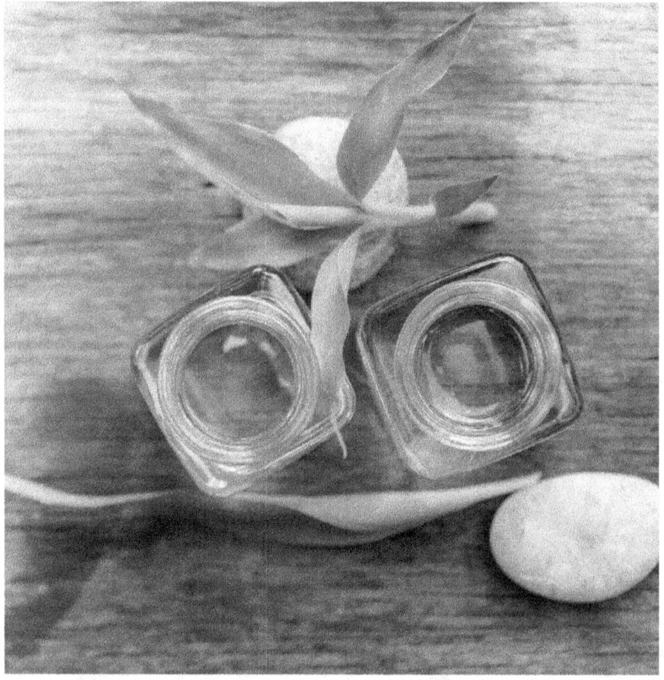

Are you looking for a natural way to improve your wellbeing?

Do you seek an opportunity to heal physical and emotional issues in a powerful, easy way?

Are you eager to learn the secrets of essential oils?

Essential oils are natural, organic compounds that have been used for thousands of years in the alternative health community. They have many potential uses, but their most popular use is to provide a wide range of health benefits.

Uncovering the Power of Essential Oils will teach you how to make the right blend to suit your specific needs and how to apply it through massage, bathing, diffusing, inhalation and more. With clear and accurate instructions, you'll be able to use essential oils correctly and safely in order to aid your overall wellbeing and positively affect your lifestyle.

- Unlock a new world of natural healing possibilities
- Understand the power of a wide variety of essential oil blends
- Learn the secrets of application, inhalation, diffusing, and aromatherapy massage
- Get the most out of your body and mind with natural remedies

Gain insight and wisdom about the power of essential oils and start your own journey towards becoming an essential oil expert.

Get your copy of Uncovering the Power of Essential Oils today.

Essential Oil Blends for Fighting Infection and Boosting Immunity

Recipe 1. Wide Awake Immunity Blend

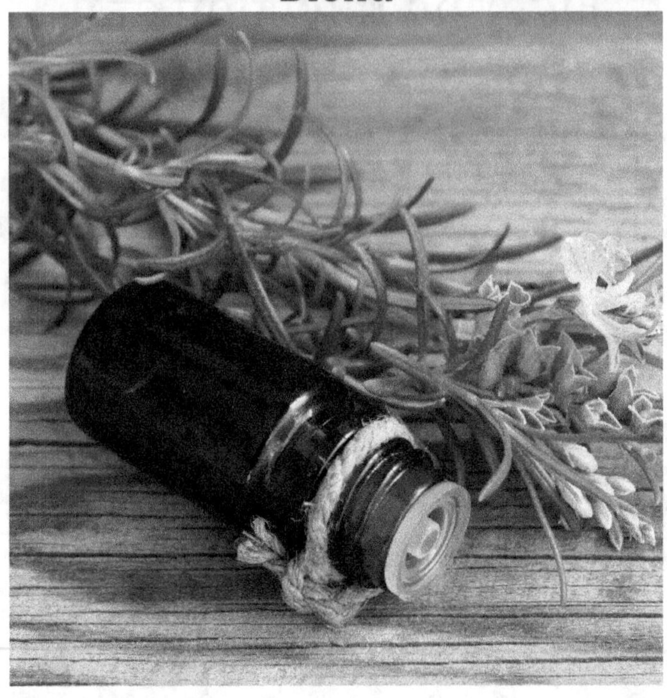

The List of Ingredients:

1. Carrier oil like jojoba, etc.
2. 1 drop of Clove oil
3. 3 drops of Rosemary oil
4. 2 drops of Cinnamon oil
5. 4 drops of Orange oil

Method:

Step 1   Pour the oils including carrier oil into a diffuser. It will offer you anti-viral and anti-bacterial properties to help fight off colds and the flu.

Step 2   Diffuse the oils for 1/2-hour intervals several times per week. Diffusing will clean your home and get rid of airborne bacteria. It's one of the most productive ways to keep your body healthy.

Recipe 2. Cleaning Spray for Supporting Immunity

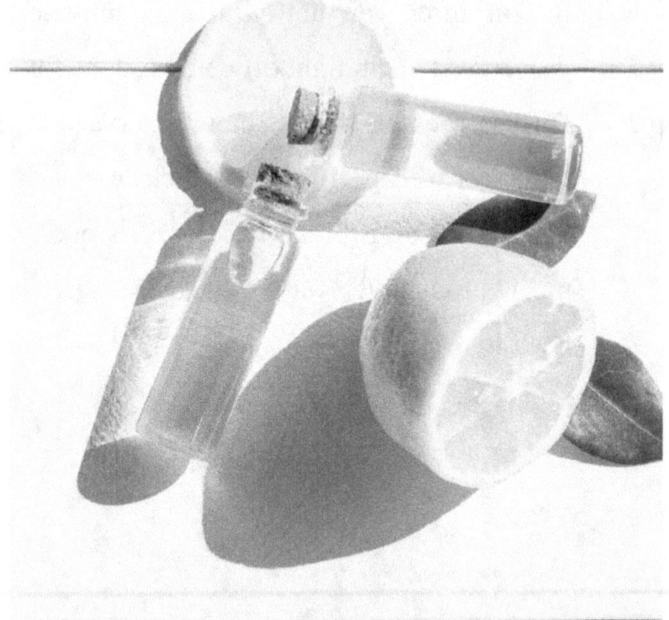

The List of Ingredients:

1. 12 drops of Cinnamon oil
2. Vinegar
3. Carrier oil
4. 12 drops of Rosemary oil
5. 12 drops of Lemon oil

Method:

Step 1   Add 4 tbsp. of vinegar to a spray bottle.

Step 2   Add essential oils and carrier oils.

Step 3   Add water and shake before you use the spray.

Recipe 3. Cold and Flu Blend

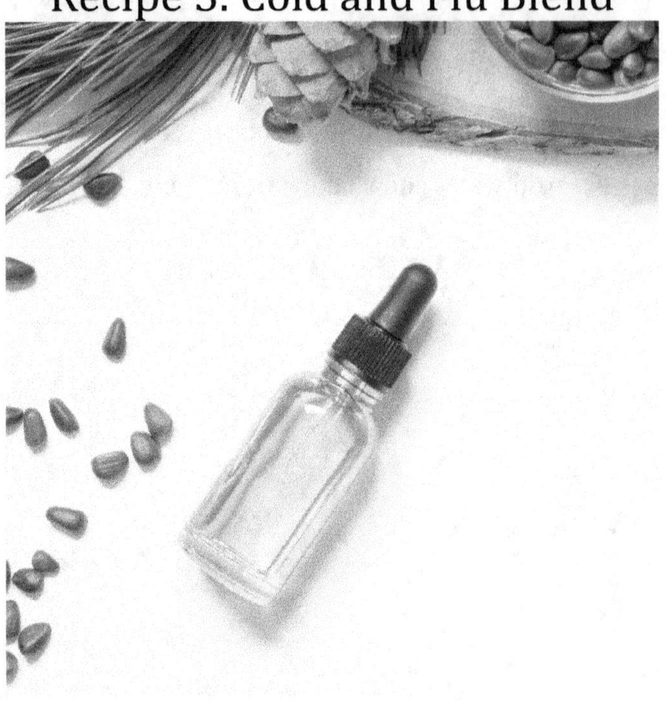

The List of Ingredients:

1. 5 drops of Tea Tree oil
2. 1 ounce of carrier oil, like jojoba, coconut, almond, etc.
3. 5 drops of Cypress oil
4. 5 drops Cedarwood oil
5. 3 drops of Lemon oil

Method:

Step 1   Add essential oils to an ounce of your favorite
           carrier oil. Apply it topically to your neck and
           chest. This solution is a 2% dilution, so you can
           use it yourself and also on kids over two years
           of age.

Recipe 4. Inhaled Immunity Boosting Blend

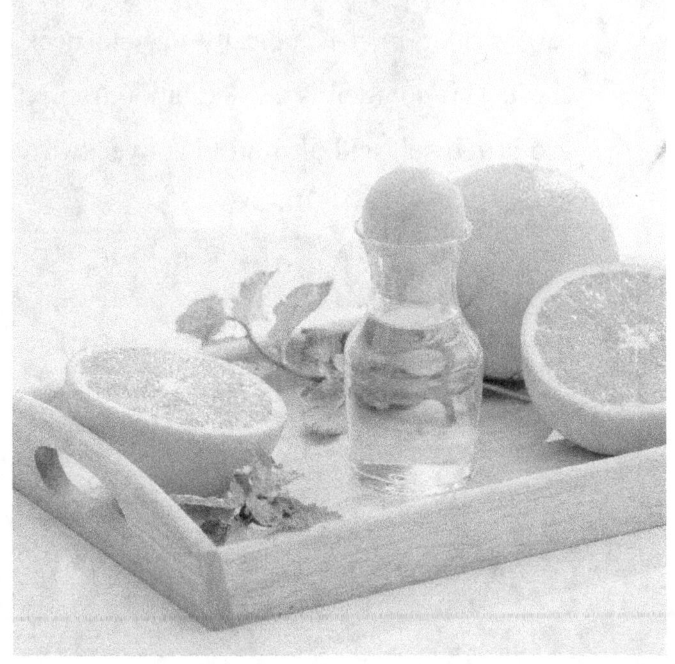

The List of Ingredients:

1. 2 or 3 drops of Orange or Rosemary oil
2. 2 cups of hot water for steam

Method:

Step 1   Add your essential oil to the steaming water in a medium basin. Use a towel to cover your head. Hold your head just above the water basin.

Close your eyes, breathe in through the nose,
and exhale through the mouth.

Recipe 5. Relaxing Immunity Support Blend

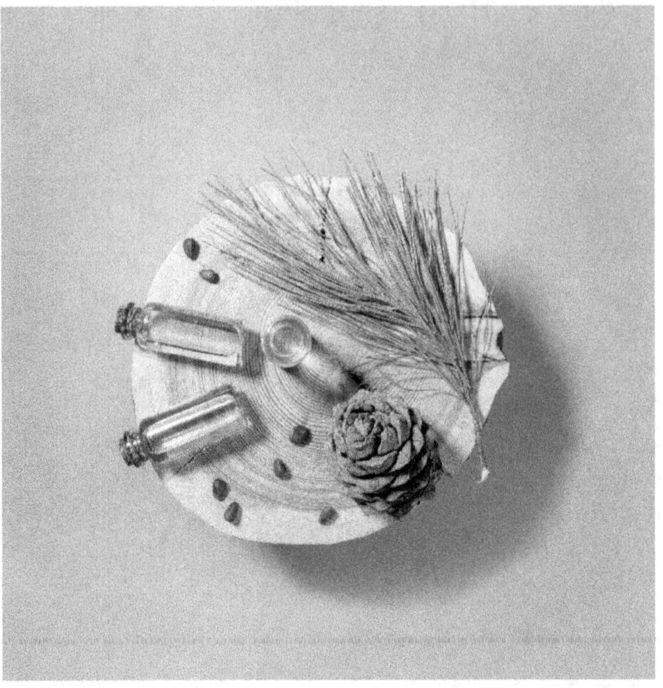

The List of Ingredients:

1.   3 drops of Cedarwood oil

2.   5 drops of Cypress essential oil

3.   1 ounce of jojoba carrier oil

4.   4 drops of Lavender oil

Method:

Step 1   Add the oils and a carrier oil to a diffuser or inhaler.

Step 2   This blend of oils, used in a diffuser, will clear the air of germs. Or, you can use it in a personal inhaler.

Step 3   You can also make a cleaning spray for countertops and doorknobs, which are often germ-ridden.

Essential Oil Blends for Alleviating Aches, Pains, Headaches, and Migraines

Recipe 6. Essential Oil Blend for Migraine Relief

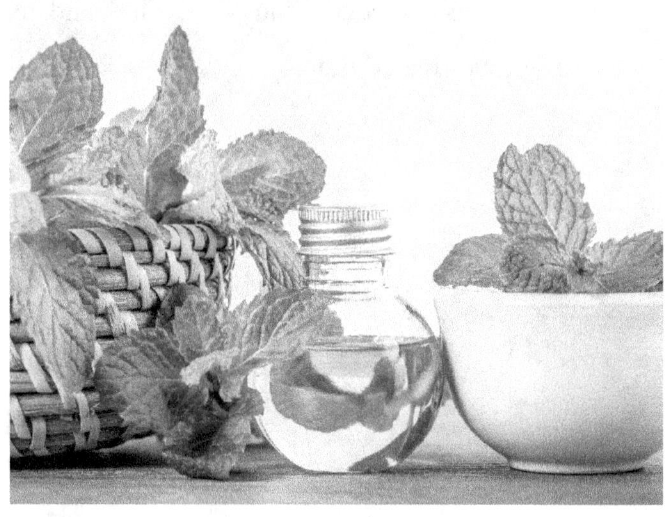

The List of Ingredients:

1. 2 drops of Lavender oil
2. 2 drops of Melissa oil
3. 2 drops of Rose oil

Method:

Step 1   Boil your kettle. Pour steaming water into a bowl. Add the essential oils.

Step 2   Place your head above the bowl with a towel over it. The towel will help in circulating the steam into your nasal passages and around your face. Breathe naturally. The steam and oils may ease the migraine somewhat, settle your mind down and relieve sinus pressure and other migraine-related issues.

Recipe 7. Arthritis Relief Essential Oil Blend

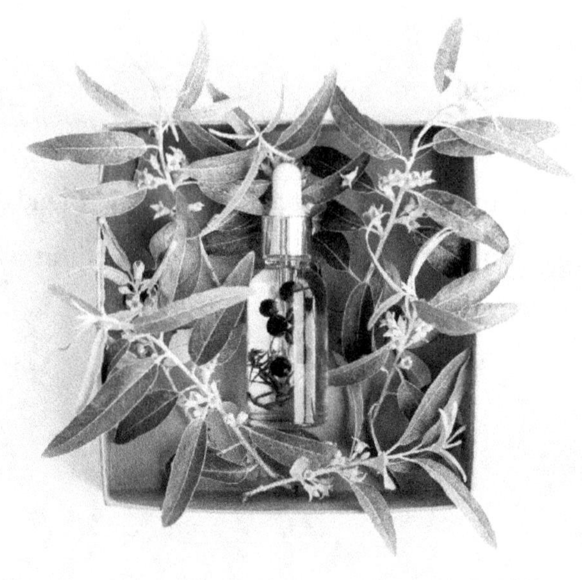

The List of Ingredients:

1. 1 oz. of apricot oil
2. 8 drops of Lavender EO
3. 4 drops of Marjoram EO
4. 1 oz. of almond oil
5. 8 drops of Eucalyptus EO
6. 4 drops of Peppermint EO
7. 2 tsp. of jojoba oil
8. 4 drops of Rosemary EO

Method:

Step 1   Combine the essential and carrier oils in a rollerball bottle.

Step 2   Apply to any joints where you experience arthritis.

Step 3   This is a very diluted and gentle blend, so you can use it multiple times a day and for extended time periods.

Recipe 8. Inflammation Relief Blend

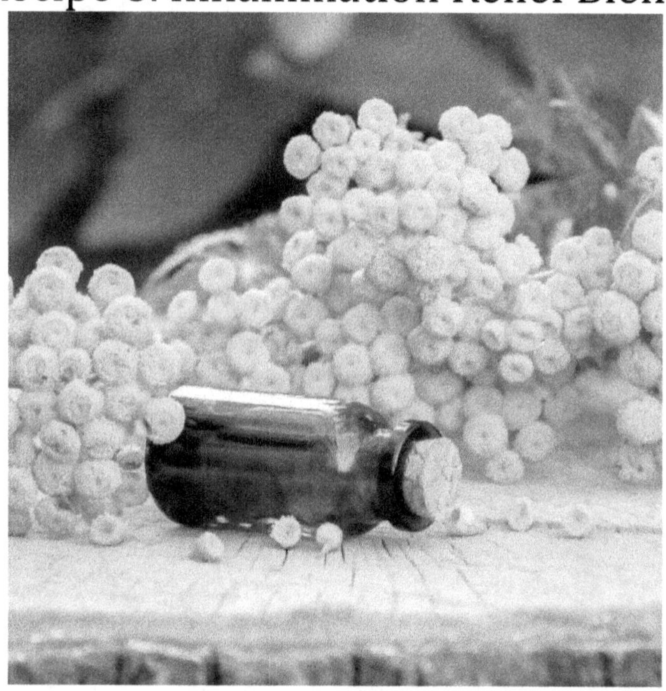

The List of Ingredients:

1. 10 drops of Eucalyptus oil

2. 30 drops of Helichrysum oil

3. 2 to 5 oz. of carrier oil – almond oil, coconut oil, jojoba, 10 drops of Peppermint oil

4. 10 drops of Spruce oil

Method:

Step 1 Add essential oils to a carrier oil in a dark-colored roller bottle.

Step 2 Allow the mixture to sit for a day before use.

Step 3 Use by applying to aching joints to help in inflammation reduction. Can be used multiple times a day.

Recipe 9. Joint Pain Relief Blend

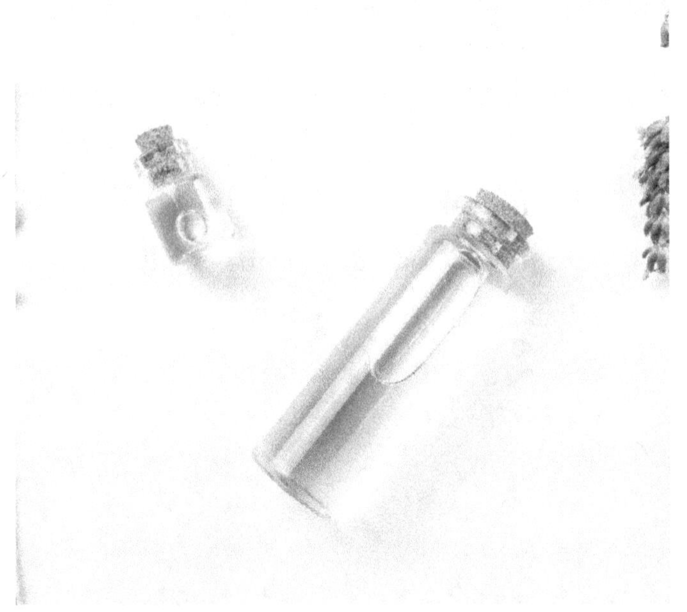

The List of Ingredients:

1. 10 drops of Lavender EO
2. 5 drops of Eucalyptus EO
3. 10 ml (1/3 ounce) of carrier oil like coconut, Argan, jojoba, etc.
4. 3 drops of Peppermint EO
5. 5 drops of Birch EO
6. 5 drops of Rosemary EO

Method:

Step 1   Add essential oils to a 10-20 ml dark-colored glass bottle with a rollerball.

Step 2   Top off the bottle with your chosen carrier oil.

Step 3   Cap the bottle. Blend gently by rolling between your palms.

Step 4   Apply when needed to stiff, swollen, or painful joints.

Recipe 10. Headache Massage Blend

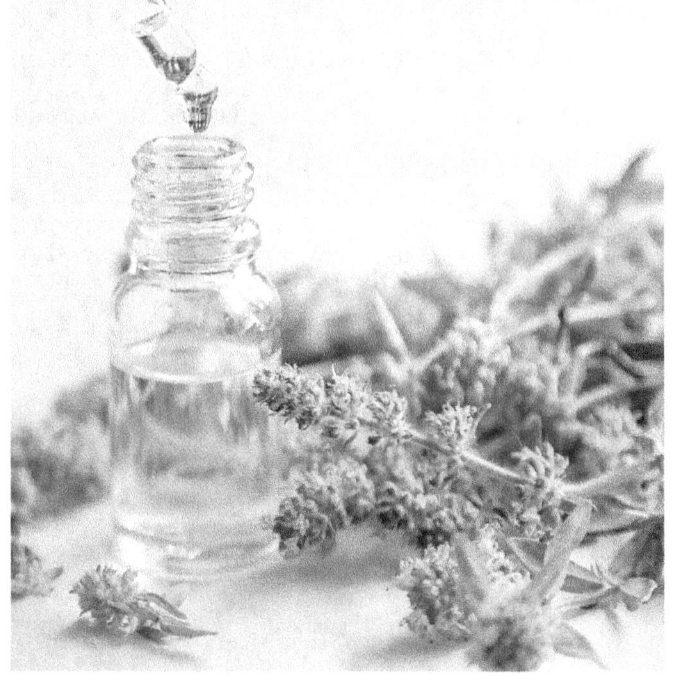

The List of Ingredients:

1. 6 to 8 drops total of Spearmint, Eucalyptus, or Peppermint oils
2. 1 ounce of carrier oil, like sweet almond or jojoba oil

Method:

Step 1   Combine the carrier oil and your essential oils in 1-ounce cobalt or amber glass bottle with a ball. Mix it by rolling the bottle gently in your hands.

Step 2   To utilize the oil, roll one to four drops on your fingers and then massage them onto the forehead, temples, or back of the neck. Be sure you don't get the oils near your eyes.

Essential Oil Blends for Balancing Hormones & Boosting Hair & Skin Health

Recipe 11. Sensitive Skin Relief Blend

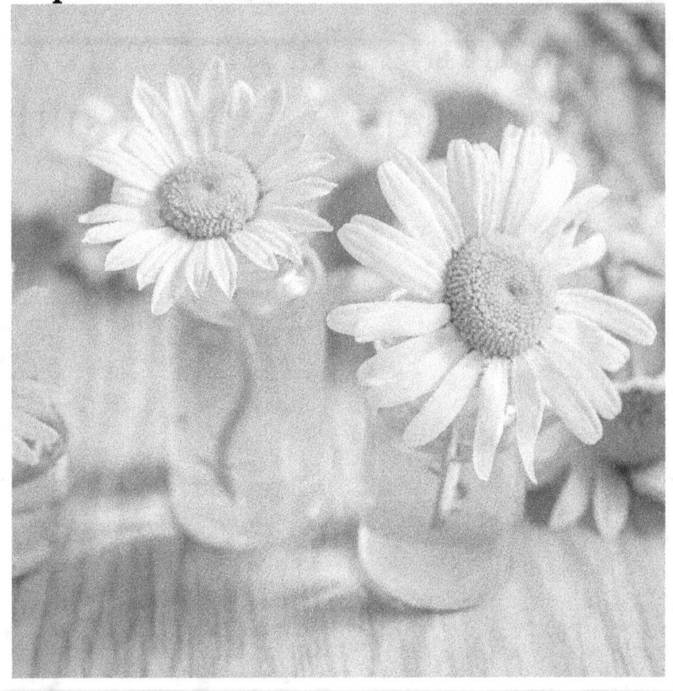

The List of Ingredients:

1. 8 drops of German Chamomile EO
2. 8 drops of Roman Chamomile EO
3. 1 tbsp. of carrier oil Hazelnut
4. 5 drops of Lavender EO
5. 9 drops of Helichrysum EO
6. 2 tbsp. of carrier oil Primrose
7. 1 tbsp. of carrier oil Musk Rose

Method:

Step 1   Mix oils in a dark-colored two-ounce bottle.

Step 2   Use on sensitive skin one or more times per day.

Step 3   Remember your skin can absorb oils more fully
           at bedtime.

Recipe 12. Hair Health Blend

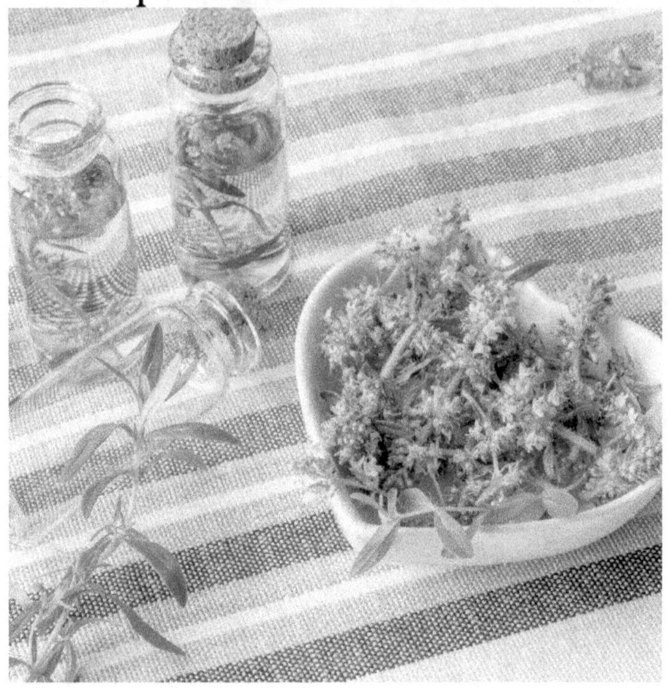

The List of Ingredients:

1. 6 drops of Peppermint oil

2. 6 drops of Rosemary oil

3. 3/8 cup of filtered water or carrier oil

Method:

Step 1   Put the carrier oil in a dark glass container with a rollerball.

Step 2   Add the essential oils.

Step 3   Place some oil blend on fingertips. Massage it
           into your scalp.

Recipe 13. Hormone Balance Blend

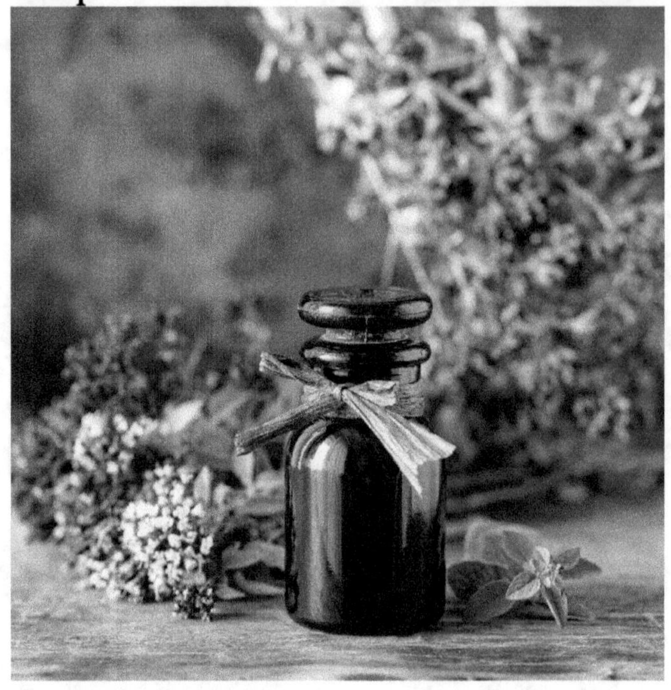

The List of Ingredients:

1.   30 drops of Ylang Ylang oil

2.   1 ounce of Evening Primrose carrier oil

3.   30 drops of Thyme oil

4.   30 drops of Clary Sage oil

Method:

Step 1   Mix oils together in 2-oz. dark-colored bottle.

Step 2   Rub five drops onto your neck two times a day.

Essential Oil Blends for Reducing Anxiety and Stress

Recipe 14. Chill Out Blend

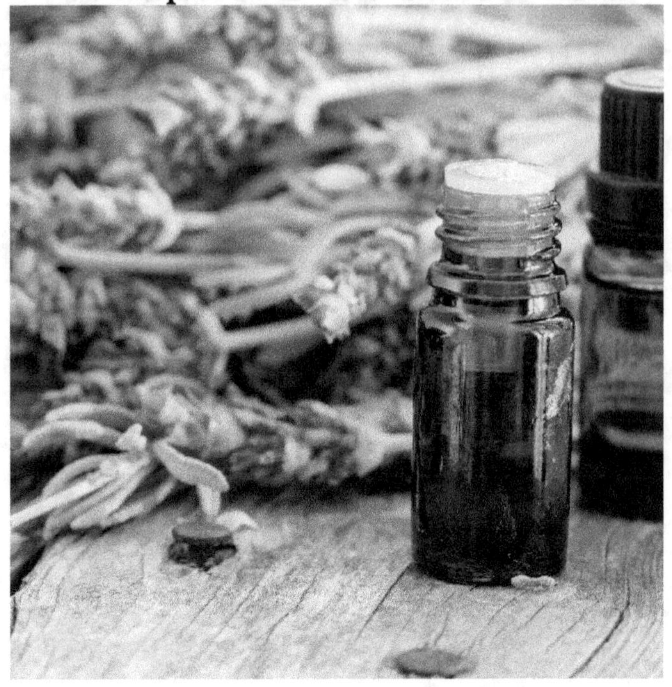

The List of Ingredients:

1. 1 drop of Clary Sage oil

2. 1 drop of Lavender oil

3. Jojoba oil or coconut oil, etc., for a carrier oil

4. 1 drop of Lemon oil

Method:

Step 1   Mix the carrier oil and essential oils in a
          diffuser. Allow it to fill a room with its relaxing
          essence.

Recipe 15. Finding a Happy Place Citrus Blend

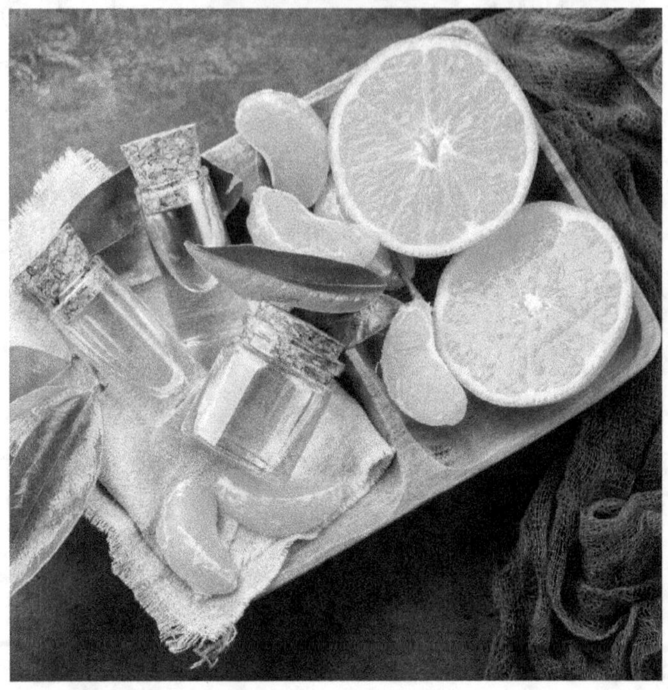

The List of Ingredients:

1. Carrier oil like coconut oil, jojoba oil, etc.

2. 2 drops of Tangerine EO

3. 2 drops of Grapefruit EO

4. 2 drops of Orange EO

Method:

Step 1   Mix oils. Use a diffuser before bedtime and
          right at bedtime.

Recipe 16. Blend for Overcoming Negative Energy

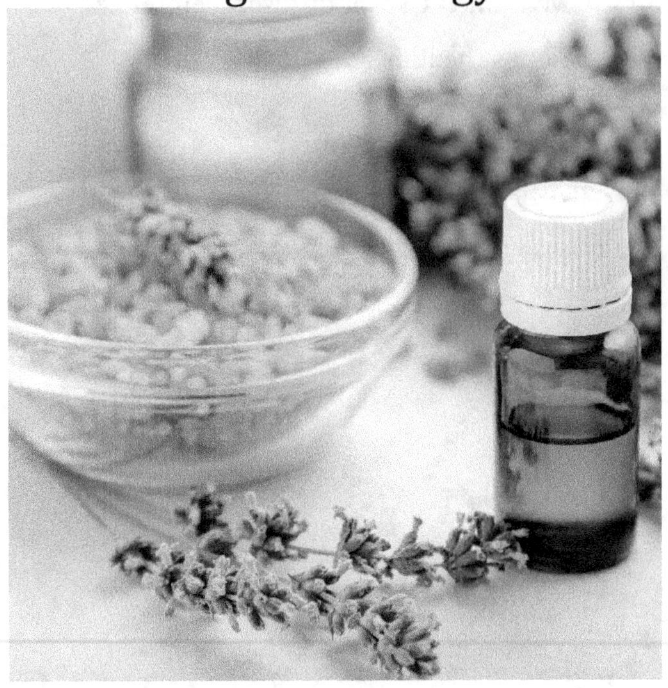

The List of Ingredients:

1. 2 drops of Ylang Ylang oil

2. 4 drops of Lavender oil

3. 2 drops of Roman Chamomile oil

Method:

Step 1   Mix oils together in a dark-colored bottle.

Step 2   Rub five drops on your wrists a couple of times
          per day.

Recipe 17. Be Happy Blend

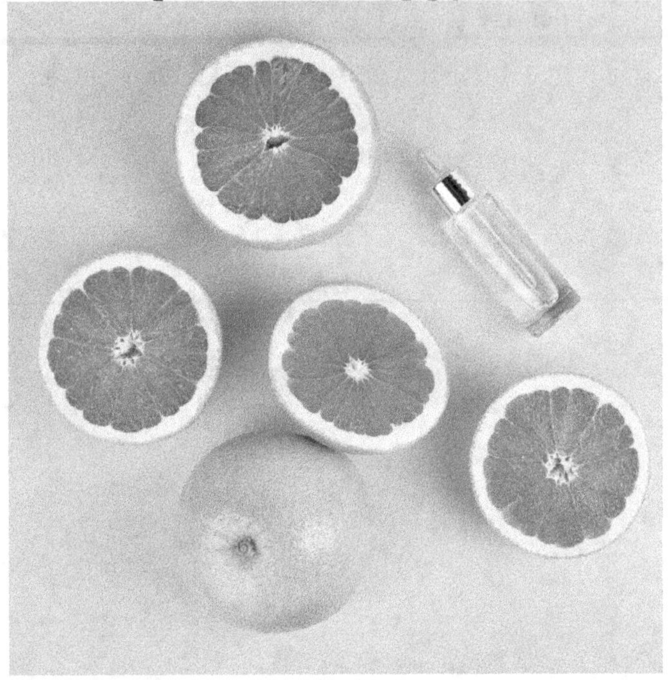

The List of Ingredients:

1. 10 drops of Roman Chamomile EO
2. 70 drops of Grapefruit EO
3. 30 drops of Sweet Orange EO
4. 20 drops of Clary Sage EO
5. 50 drops of Lavender EO

Method:

Step 1   Combine your oils in an amber glass bottle. Swirl and mix the oils. Store in a cool place out of direct sunlight when you're not using it.

Step 2   To use in a diffuser: Pour oil blend into the diffuser and turn it on for 1/2-hour intervals and off for 1-hour intervals.

Step 3   To use in a roll-on bottle: follow step 1 and use on your chest, the back of your neck, and the bottoms of your feet.

Recipe 18. Reset after an Anxious Day Blend

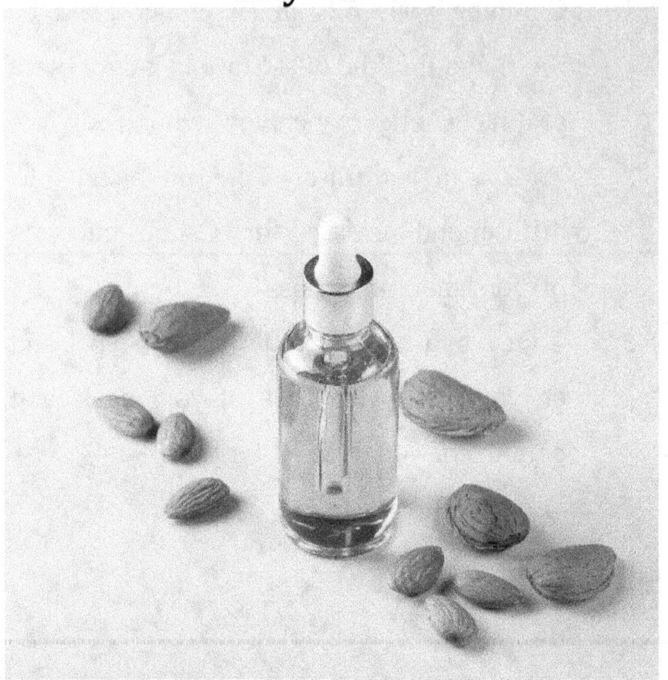

The List of Ingredients:

1. 2 drops of Clary Sage EO

2. Almond carrier oil

3. 1 drop of Patchouli EO

4. 2 drops of Geranium EO

5. 1 drop of Ylang Ylang EO

Method:

Step 1   Add 30 EO drops to a 10-ML bottle with a rollerball. Fill the rest of the room with the almond carrier oil. Roll into temples, feet, wrists, and the back of your neck.

Step 2   You can also add the oils to a cool-air, ultrasonic diffuser.

Essential Oil Blends for Helping to Get Restful Sleep

Recipe 19. Dreamland Blend

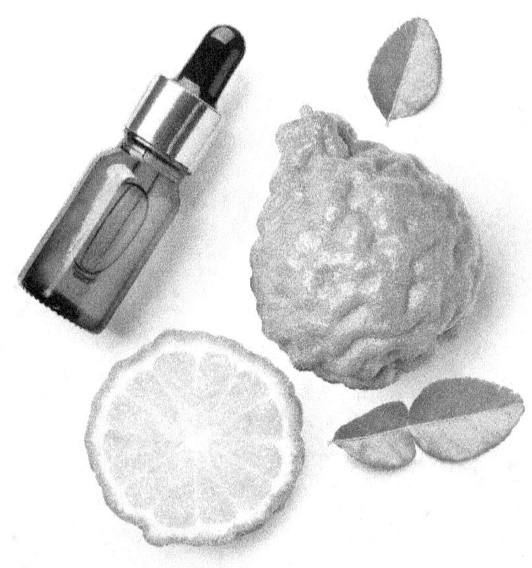

The List of Ingredients:

1. 2 drops of Bergamot oil

2. Jojoba or coconut oil, etc., as a carrier oil

3. 1 drop of Vetiver oil

4. 1 drop of Patchouli oil

Method:

Step 1   Mix the essential oils with your favorite carrier
         oil and use in a diffuser near your bed.

Recipe 20. Cedarwood Sleep Remedy

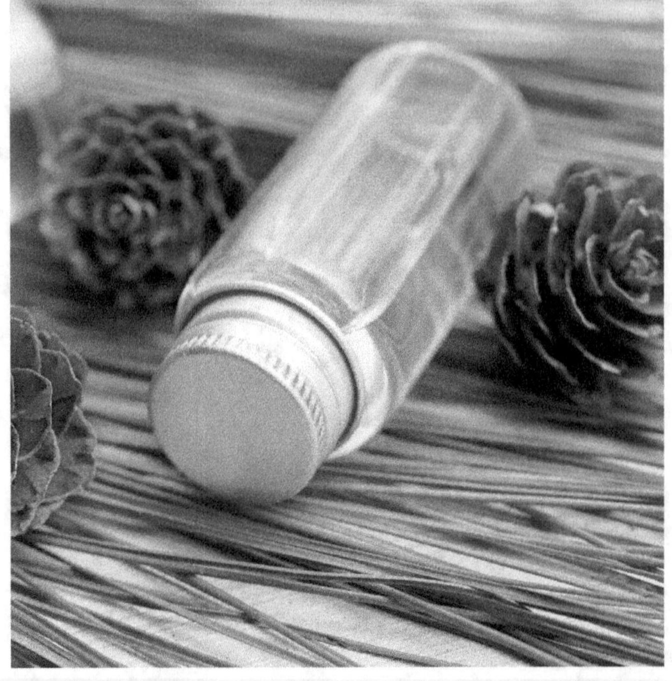

The List of Ingredients:

1. 1 drop of Lavender oil
2. 1 drop of Marjoram oil
3. 1 drop of Cedarwood oil

Method:

Step 1   Combine your oils in a diffuser. Add water as recommended by the company that manufactured the diffuser.

Step 2   Turn the diffuser on beside the bed 15-20 minutes before you go to bed. It will create a more restful environment that helps you doze into sleep more readily.

Recipe 21. Stress-Free Sleep

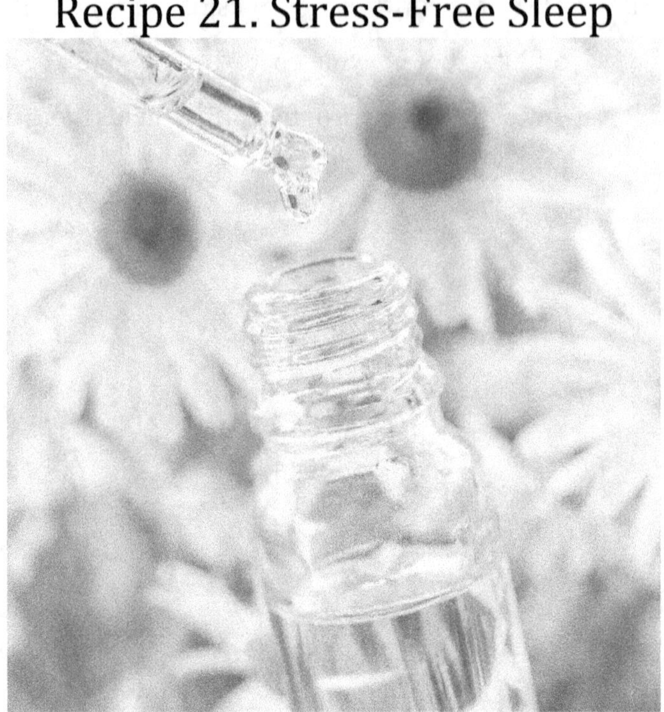

The List of Ingredients:

1. 2 drops of Sweet Marjoram EO
2. 2 drops of Lavender EO
3. 4 drops of Roman Chamomile EO

Method:

Step 1   For a diffuser: Fill with filtered water to fill the line. Add the essential oils. Diffuse for about 20 minutes before bedtime and continue 1/2 hour after you go to bed.

Step 2   For a bath soak: Double the recipe. Add that blend along with 2 tbsp. of coconut oil and 1 cup of Epsom salts to a warm bath, with water still running. Soak in the wonderful blend for 20 minutes to a half-hour.

Recipe 22. Lavender-and-More Sleep Blend

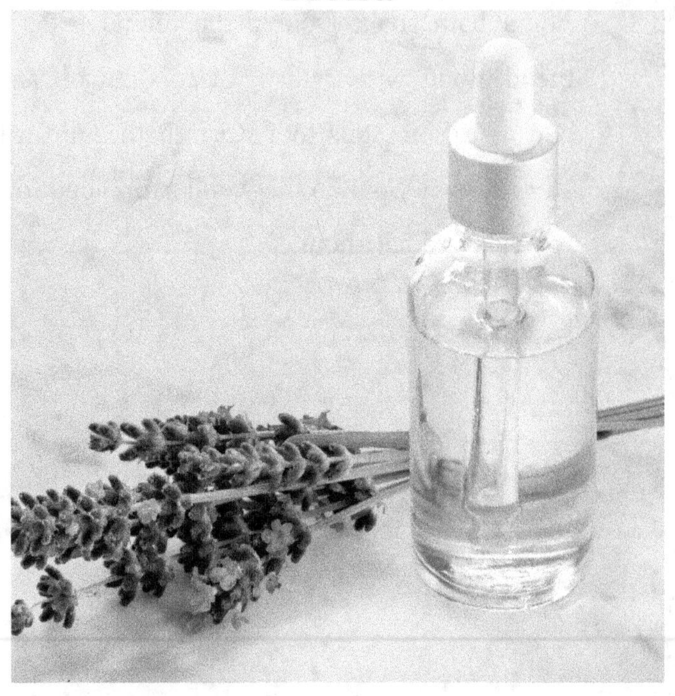

The List of Ingredients:

1. 2 drops of Cedarwood EO

2. 2 drops of Orange EO

3. Carrier oil

4. 4 drops of Lavender EO

5. 2 drops of Ylang Ylang EO

Method:

Step 1   Fill your diffuser using filtered water to the designated line. Add essential oil blend.

Step 2   Essential Oil Blends for Improving Brain Function These recipes were designed to help in enhancing memory retention and concentration. When you select and use essential oils, follow the safety precautions noted in the introduction and online. Remember, while essential oils can be helpful, they are not a valid substitute for actual medical care.

Recipe 23. Concentration Enhancement Blend

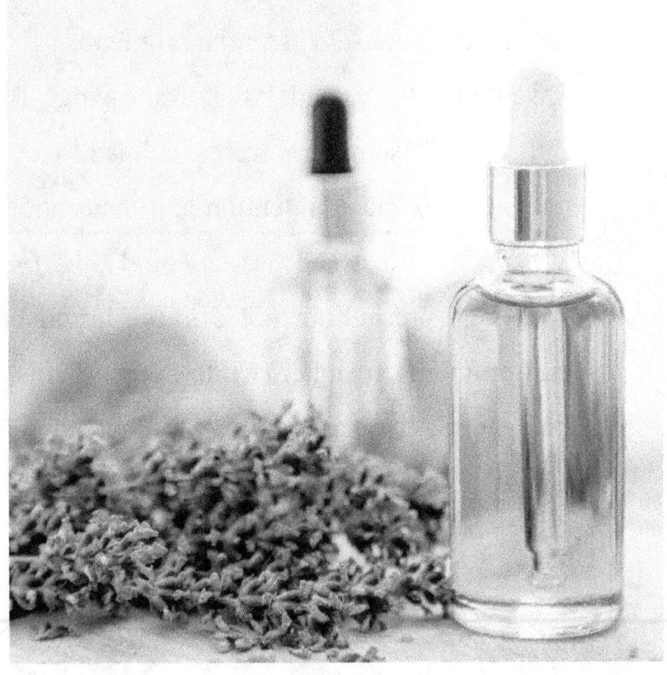

The List of Ingredients:

1. Carrier oil of choice
2. 1 drop Spearmint oil
3. 3 drops Rosemary oil
4. 3 drops Geranium oil
5. 4 drops Lavender oil
6. 2 drops Tangerine oil

Method:

Step 1   Blend your oils carefully. Add a carrier oil.

Step 2   Massage the blend into temples if you want to
use it topically or apply with a rollerball to the
back of the neck or soles of the feet.

Step 3   If you want to treat a room where you study, use
a diffuser.

Recipe 24. Memory Boosting Blend

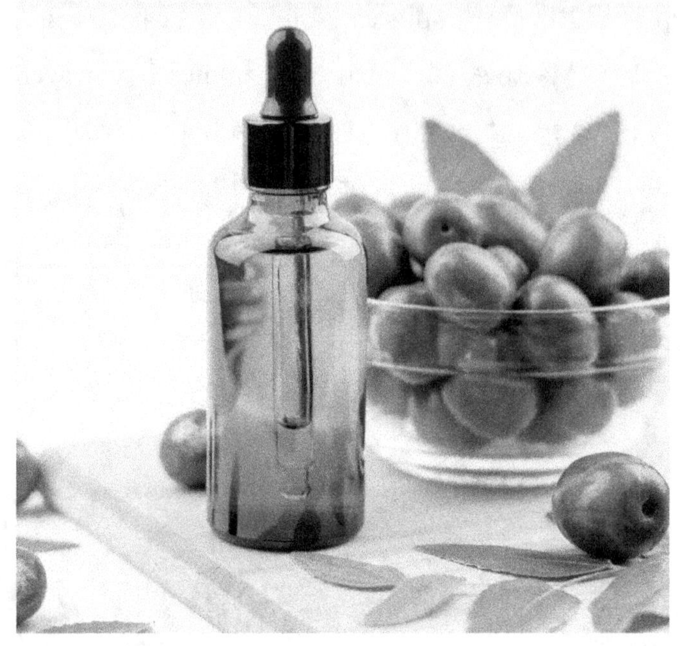

The List of Ingredients:

1. 2 drops of Lavender EO
2. 2 drops of Rosemary EO
3. 2 drops of Eucalyptus EO
4. 8 drops of carrier oil like coconut oil, jojoba, etc.

Method:

Step 1   Dilute the essential oils using your carrier oil.

Step 2   Pour the oils into a dark-colored bottle with a
          rollerball top.

Step 3   Test your skin to make sure the area you will
          massage is not over-sensitive to the oils.

Step 4   Massage onto your forehead and the back of
          your neck.

Recipe 25. Clear Mind Blend

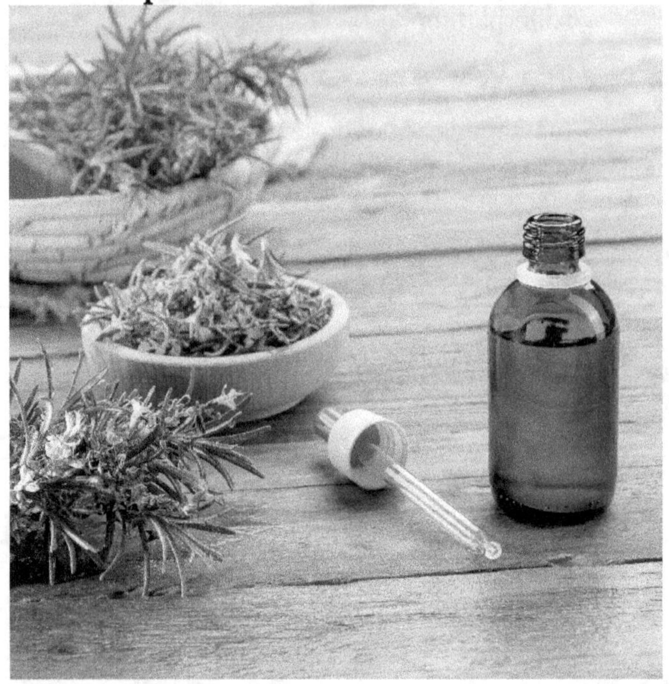

The List of Ingredients:

1. 2 drops of Rosemary oil

2. 2 drops of Cypress oil

3. Carrier oil of your choice

4. 1 drop of Basil oil

Method:

Step 1   Multiply the oil blend by four. This will give you 20 total drops. Add these oils to a glass bottle of a dark color. Roll in your hands to mix.

Step 2   If using a diffuser, use the instructions from the manufacturer of your chosen model and brand to mix the blend in the diffuser.

Essential Oil Blends for Helping with Depression

Recipe 26. Mood Lifting Blend

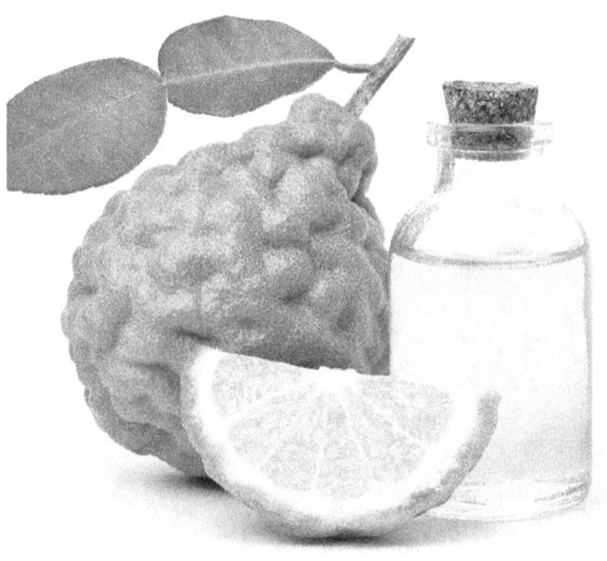

The List of Ingredients:

1. 10 drops of Bergamot oil EO
2. 1 drop of Ylang Ylang EO
3. Carrier oil of choice
4. 1 drop of Geranium oil EO
5. 5 drops of Grapefruit oil EO
6. 4 drops of Orange oil EO

Method:

Step 1   When you blend these oils, they are often put into inhalers. You can carry them in a bag or leave one in your car, to help with road rage. Use this blend when you need an uplifting feeling.

Recipe 27. Ease Depression Mood Blend

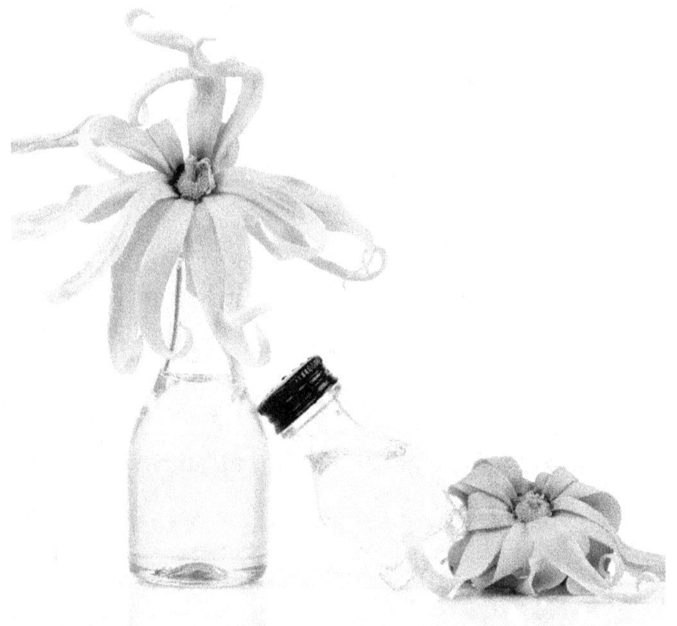

The List of Ingredients:

1. 20 drops of Sweet Orange EO
2. 20 drops of Peppermint EO
3. 20 drops of Lemon EO
4. 20 drops of Lavender EO
5. Carrier of choice
6. 20 drops of Ylang Ylang EO
7. 10 drops of Patchouli EO

Method:

Step 1   Add 20 drops of each of your essential oils above to a ceramic bowl. Stir.

Step 2   Use a dropper from an amber bottle to pick up and transfer oils into the bottle.

Step 3   Add carrier oil. Close bottle. Shake well.

Step 4   For the diffuser, add six to eight drops to a cold-air-based diffuser. Allow it to run for about 15 minutes per day. While you take in the scents, you can think about nothing, or meditate. The aroma will ease your mind and body, creating positive energy.

Step 5   When you use this as a bath blend, these oils will relax the soul and improve the mood. Mix 10 to 15 drops of this blend with a cup of Epsom salts. Add it to a just-drawn hot bath and allow it to disperse. Soak in the tub and let relaxation overtake you for 20-25 minutes.

Step 6   To make a mist to create a happy room, pour a half-cup of filtered water into a dark glass spray bottle. Add 20 drops of the blend above. Close the bottle and then shake. Spray the room.

Step 7   Roller bottles work so well because you can take them with you. Add 25 drops of the blend above into a bottle with a roller. Top it up with carrier oil. Roll on ends of hair, shoulder, collarbones, and wrists as desired. It will help in boosting your mood.

Recipe 28. Citrus Bergamot Depression Blend

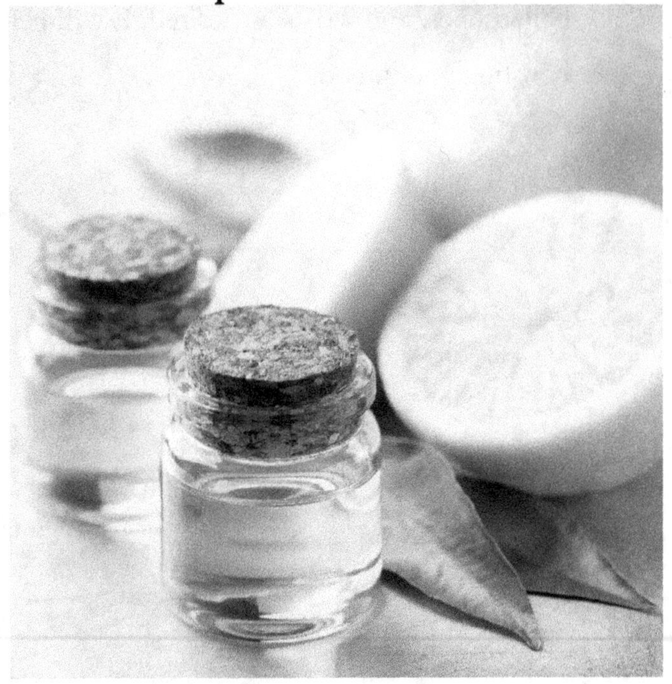

The List of Ingredients:

1. 5 drops Clary Sage oil
2. 10 drops Lavender oil
3. 5 drops Grapefruit oil
4. Your favorite carrier oil
5. 5 drops Bergamot oil
6. 10 drops Orange oil

Method:

Step 1   Add the essential oils to a roller bottle. Fill the remainder with a carrier oil. Carrier oils are quite important, particularly if your skin tends to be sensitive.

Step 2   Apply as needed to the neck, wrists, or feet.

Recipe 29. Peace of Mind Blend

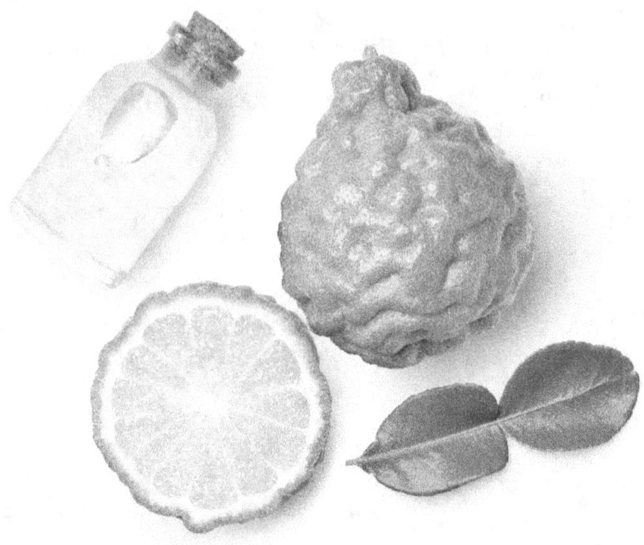

The List of Ingredients:

1. 20 drops of Bergamot EO
2. Carrier oil, like jojoba, etc.
3. 4 drops Lavender EO
4. 4 drops of Clary Sage EO

Method:

Step 1   Use a dropper to add essential oil to bottles with rollers.

Step 2	Top with the jojoba oil and gently shake.

Step 3	Roll on your palms and rub them together. Inhale the scent. Rub the blend on your forehead, back of the neck, behind the ears, and on your temples.

Step 4	Cup your hands. Hold them over your nose. Take several moments to breathe in their benefits.

Recipe 30. Anxiety-Based Depression Blend

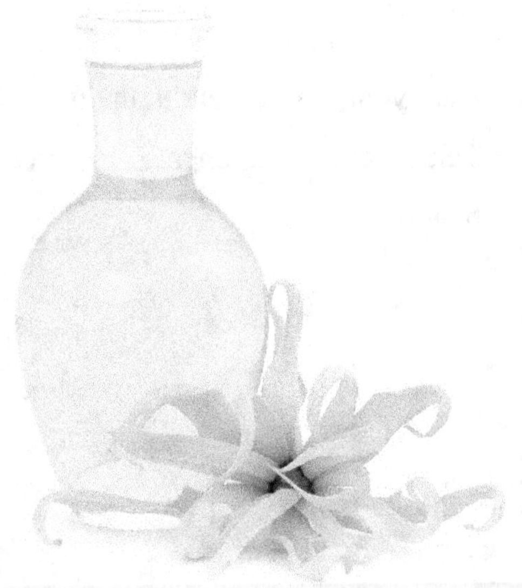

The List of Ingredients:

1. 10 drops Ylang Ylang oil
2. 5 drops Chamomile oil
3. 5 drops Frankincense oil
4. 5 drops Sandalwood oil
5. 10 drops Lavender oil
6. Your favorite carrier oil

Method:

Step 1   Add essential oils to a rollerball bottle.

Step 2   Fill the bottle with a carrier oil.

Step 3   Apply to your neck, wrists, or feet.

Essential Oil Blends for Boosting Energy Levels

Recipe 31. Get Yourself Going Blend

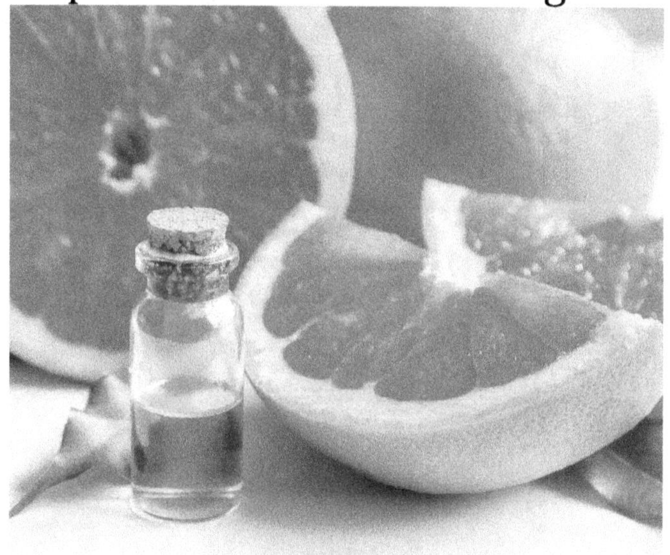

The List of Ingredients:

1. 2 drops of Grapefruit oil
2. Your carrier oil of choice
3. 1 drop of Peppermint oil
4. 1 drop of Lime oil

Method:

Step 1   Add essential oils plus water to the diffuser. Check the instructions your manufacturer sent about using distilled water, etc.

Recipe 32. Energizing Blend

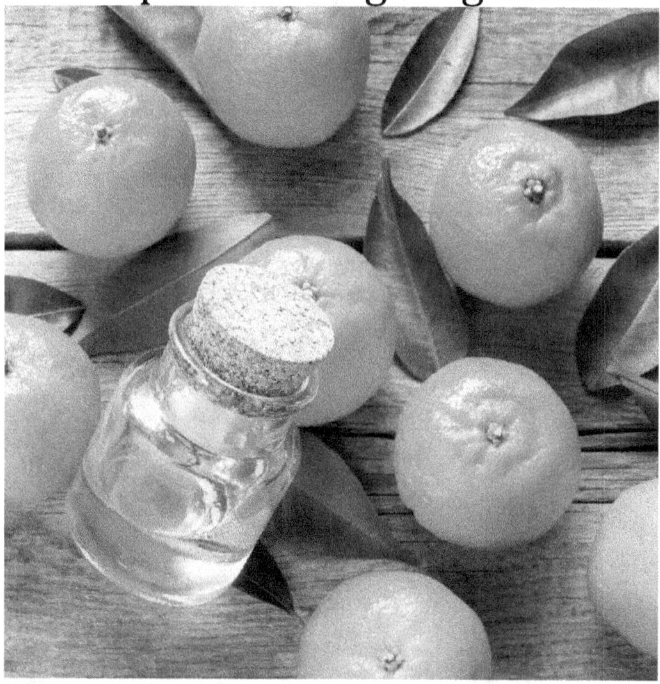

The List of Ingredients:

1. 1 drop of Thyme oil
2. 3 drops of Tangerine oil

Method:

Step 1   Pour the essential oils into your diffuser and enjoy the results.

Recipe 33. Essential Oil Blend to Fight Fatigue

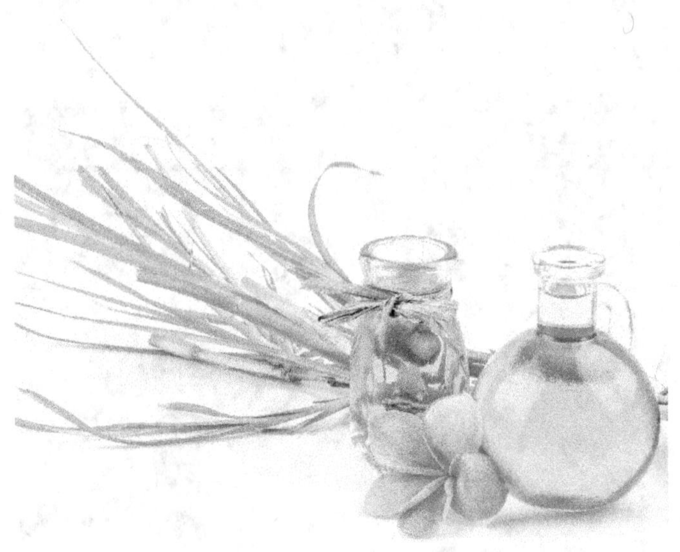

The List of Ingredients:

1. 1 drop of Rosemary oil

2. 1 drop of Eucalyptus oil

3. 1 drop of Lemongrass oil

Method:

Step 1   Add essential oils and the proper amount of water into your diffuser. Refer to your owner's manual to determine whether you need to use distilled or filtered water.

Step 2   Essential Oil Blends Aiding in Proper Digestion
No one likes to discuss digestive issues in public. That means when we have them, we must suffer in silence. There are many people who have gastrointestinal problems today, causing more visits to hospitals and clinics. Lifestyle changes and OTC remedies can help, and so can the use of essential oils.

Recipe 34. Stomach Soothing Blend

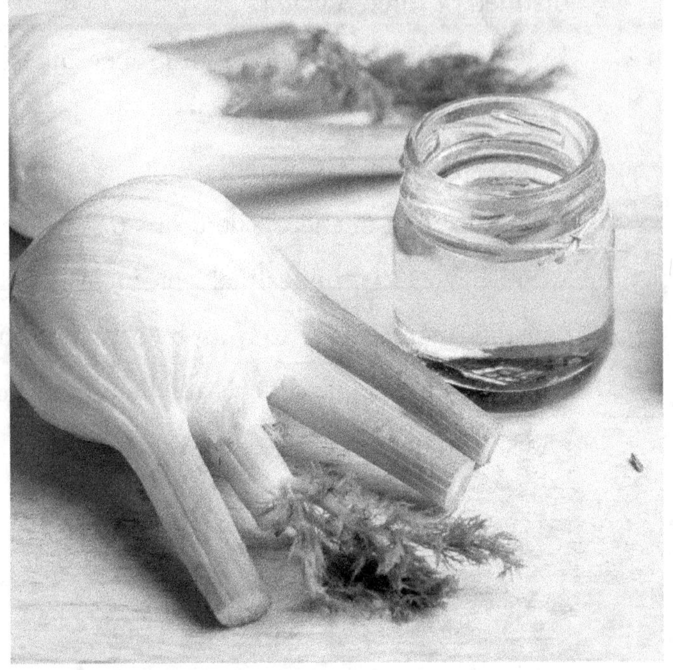

The List of Ingredients:

1. 12 drops of Fennel EO
2. 8 drops of Peppermint EO
3. 2 tbsp. of castor carrier oil
4. 10 drops of Chamomile EO

Method:

Step 1   Measure the castor oil into a tinted glass bottle. If you want it in a rollerball bottle, reduce your recipe by 1/3.

Step 2   Add essential oils.

Step 3   Store in a dry, cool place, out of direct sunlight.

Step 4   To use, place several drops on your fingers and massage them onto your stomach. You can also apply it directly to your stomach with a roller bottle.

Step 5   Massage in a clockwise direction, which is the direction in which food and drink move through your large intestine. Start close to your navel and work gradually outward.

Step 6   Begin with the pressure that is very gentle. Increase it gradually as long as it is still comfortable for you.

Step 7   Ensure that you complete five to 10 full rotations for the best effect.

Step 8   If you have a severely upset stomach, lie on your back and do the massaging for a longer time.

Step 9   Shake the bottle before you use it. Since castor oil may stain clothing, be careful that it doesn't touch any of your clothes if you are worried about staining.

Recipe 35. Stomach Pain Relief Blend

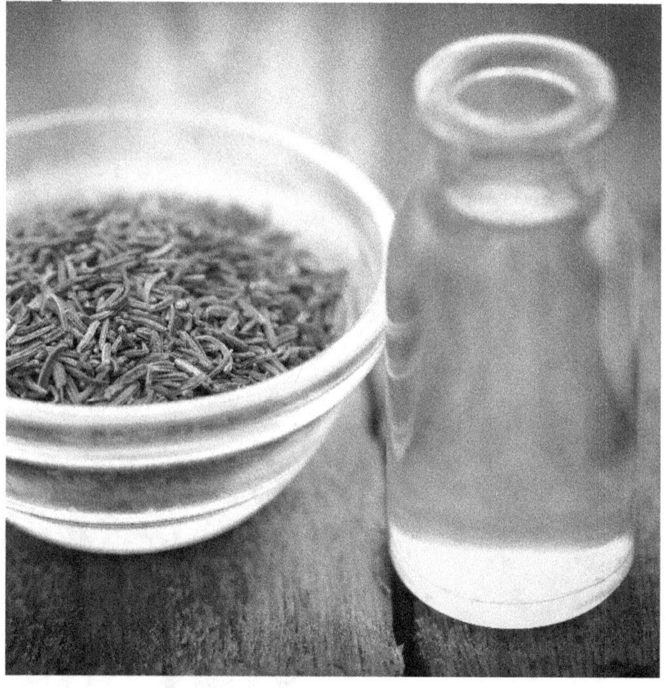

The List of Ingredients:

1. 15 drops of Cumin oil
2. 1 ounce of John's wort oil
3. 1 ounce of almond oil
4. 15 drops of Basil oil

Method:

Step 1   Mix oils. Shake before using.

Step 2   Apply oil to the stomach and massage two or
three times per day.

Essential Oil Blends for Reducing Toxicity

Recipe 36. Chemical-Free Insect Repellant Blend

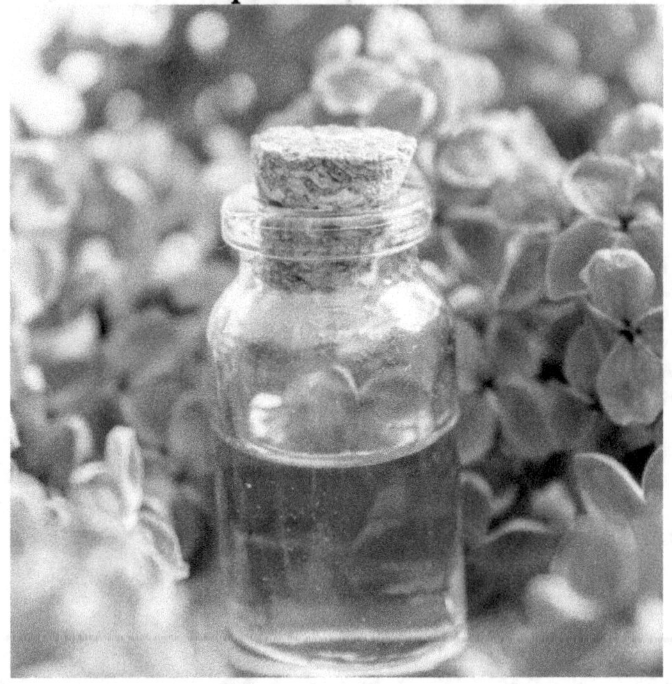

The List of Ingredients:

1. 5 drops Geranium oil
2. 5 drops Lavender oil
3. 8 ounces of water, filtered
4. 15 drops Purify oil
5. 1 x 8-ounce spray top glass bottle
6. 5 drops Cedarwood oil
7. 1/4 tsp. of non-fragrance Epsom Salt

Method:

Step 1   Place ingredients in a bottle. Shake gently to combine.

Step 2   Spray every 1-2 hours or when you need it. You can spray bugs with it, too, and kill them directly.

Recipe 37. Blend to Reduce the Toxic Load on your Body

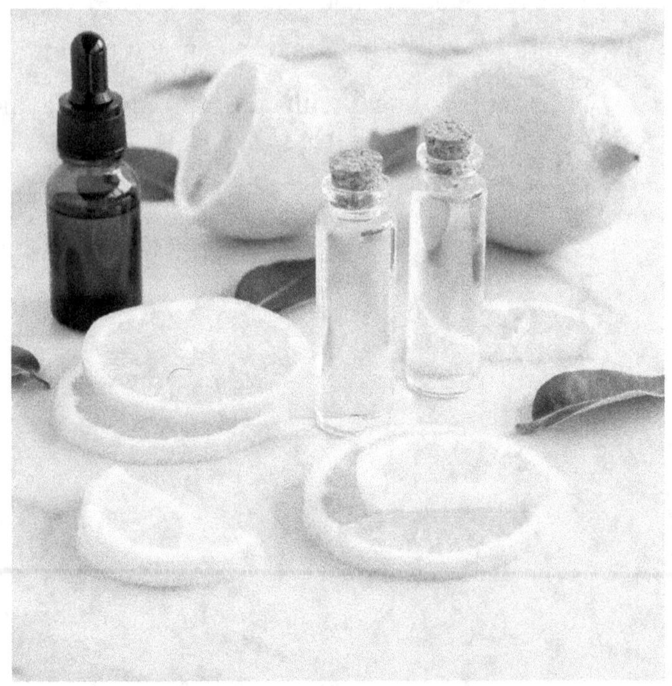

The List of Ingredients:

1. Carrier oil of your choice
2. 2 drops Geranium oil
3. 5 drops Lavender oil
4. 5 drops Lemon oil

Method:

Step 1   Place essential oils in a dark-colored glass
           bottle. Add carrier oil to fill. Shake gently.
           Spray as needed.